This is a collection of three books by Dolley Sen

Book one

THE BOOK OF TORN UP SUICIDE NOTES

Book two

THE MAENAD ANGEL POETICS

Book Three

ECCENTRIC FISH

Logos & Insanity

I first met Dolly when I was organizing a poetry festival in a squatted church where I lived in Amsterdam. She had posted a note on 'Litkicks' asking about gigs and venues in Europe, this was sent to me and I eventually asked her to come over for the festival that I was organizing in a squatted church in the heart of Amsterdam.

She arrived loaded down with books and looking very nervous. The reason why, I was to find out later, she had never performed on stage before and was having 2nd thoughts. By this time I was dealing with hoards of poets, musicians, squatters and the logistics of feeding and bedding all these people.
When at last it was her turn to read, I and the audience were not disappointed, although still extremely nervous she managed to hold their attention with her original insights that her poetry conveyed.
 Since then I have watched her turn from a nervous little poet into a roaring lioness.

We have since worked together many time around Europe and the UK, and each time I see her perform or I read her work I still get the same tingle that I got when she first performed in that old ruined church in Amsterdam.

We have become firm friends, shared tears and laughter, Pain and sorrow both through her poetry and through or lives.

All I really have to say, is that if this book is only half as good as all her others, the I and he other readers are in for a treat once more, as she takes us through a rollercoaster ride along that fine line that

borders Madness & Sanity, And if as she often states,
she is as mad as a hatter, then let madness rule supreme,
because if this is madness, then I want some of it !

Barry Fitton

Amsterdam 2007

Author of 'I Left No Footsteps Behind Me', 'Erotology'
& 'Amsterdam Nights'

THE BOOK OF TORN UP SUICIDE NOTES

By

Dolly Sen

Published by:
Chipmukapublishing
PO Box 6872
Brentwood
Essex
CM13 1ZT
United Kingdom

www.chipmunkapublishing.com

Image by Magali Moreau

DOLLY SEN BIOG

Dolly Sen was born on 23rd October 1970 in London, where she still lives.

"I had my first psychotic experience aged 14 and stopped going to school. A series of dead end jobs followed. Pretty early on I decided I didn't want any more of the 9-5 shit and spoon race, and began to write… and maybe watch 70s cop shows."

Dolly Sen is a writer, director, artist, film-maker, poet, performer, raconteur, playwright, mental health consultant, music-maker and public speaker. Since her much-acclaimed book 'The World is Full of Laughter' was published by Chipmunka in 2002, she has had 3 further books published, had a succession of performance roles around Europe and places like The Young Vic, Trafalgar Square and The Royal Festival Hall; did a poetry tour and won a poetry award from Andrew Motion; directed two plays and several films, appeared on TV, and has done spoken word at City Hall and Oxford University.

This is staggering since she dropped out of school at 14 and has no formal qualifications. She has also had to share her life with severe mental health problems. She was told she would never amount to anything but would end up in jail or Broadmoor and she believed this and was on her way there when she changed her belief into the one of believing she could do anything she wanted to do.

This proves that the mind is an amazing thing; it can drive you mad and inspire you in the same breath. And that you can do anything if you believe you can do it.

Q

Dinner queue in the psych ward
I'm stuck between 2 Jesuses
I can see they're both contemplating
feeding the 5 thousand by doing a
miracle of multiplication with the
rubbery macaroni cheese
A schizophrenic soul abuses
any god that is listening
The catatonic philosophises
with empty words
The anorexic looks down her
nose at us for indulging in
the depravity of sustenance
Why am I here?
Reality, sanity is a book of
lies, I've lost my page
I've become celestially illiterate
Because I know the ending – no
happily ever after
just lonely death
following
a life
that is just a queue
waiting, waiting
for the
madness to end

THE PARK BENCH

Everyone's a fucking philosopher.

But there's not much else to do sitting on a park bench.

And you can always tell where the most prolific philosophers sit to chew the fat. The rickety benches they preside over are cordoned off from public use by a circlet of rusting lager empties.

The way I see it: how can you philosophise and not drink yourself stupid after?

Philosophy: the investigation of the nature of being – an ultimately boring and futile subject – but it does help to pass the time.

Shithead, my fellow drinker/thinker, said philosophy is the wisdom of fools. Pretty deep, huh? As deep as the shit we are all in.

"What's the use of a philosophy degree?" Shithead once bemoaned, "It's bloody useless, in it? I mean, it doesn't pay the bills, and there is no world peace because of it, right?"

"I guess you're right," I agreed tepidly.

"Of course I'm right. Learning about philosophy is like learning to swim in set concrete."

Shithead and I discussed and argued and criticised all sorts of theories as much as our diminishing sobriety would allow. Maybe it is the drink that influences my only solid conclusion: my only handy household hint in dealing with onthological insecurity is: stay pissed. Shithead agrees with me wholeheartedly.

Why is Shithead called Shithead? Now that is an easy question to answer. I – and most of our mutual confederates – called him Shithead because that was what he was. It wasn't meant in a derogative sense – he was called much worse by the two beautiful people who brought him into this world. It was an affectionate term because we wanted to call him much worse but didn't. According to reliable sources, Shithead was one odoriferous bastard – an unblocked toilet was a bed of roses compared. When tramps and winos comment disparagingly on someone else's body odour… fucking hell… I wouldn't know personally, mind you – I lost my sense of smell through repeated punches to the nose. I think that was why we were best mates, what with me being the only person able to physically sit next to him. He smelled like shit and looked like shit. If you placed one of those plastic red lips and a fucked up, moth-eaten blond wig on a pile of shit, you'd get a fair resemblance of the human being he is. But he is an okay kind of shit… most of the time.

But inevitably the more you drink, the more of an obnoxious megalomaniac you become: you become critical of everyone and everything. You begin to think everyone is an arsehole except for you. Which is bullshit, of course. Everyone in the world is an arsehole including yourself.

Shithead is in one of those moods right now. There's supposed to be a tentative camaraderie between drunks, which is crap. It's just that we're so pissed we can't be arsed to get up and move on.

Shithead is telling me why he chooses not to be part of society. I'm not really listening; I am more intrigued by the fact that a strand of dried egg yolk in his stubble is turning green.

"If you don't make yourself available to duplicity," he went on, "society loses interest in you, it has no use for you. And you will notice if it has no use for you, you worth goes down. For example, a customer who knows the cons and psychological tricks of an unscrupulous salesperson and isn't taken in by them loses his worth in the eyes of the salesperson. That insincere smile begins to twitch and the welcoming open arms want to beat the shit out of you…"

I sit there and listen to him ramble interminably on. Thank God I only have limited access to full consciousness at the moment, which is a help in any situation, which is a fucking lifesaver, actually.

"All women are whores," Was now the subject of his morbid attention.

Here we go again, I thought.

"Why are all the women I go out with whores?"

"Maybe you specifically pick whorish women to go out with so you can say all women are whores."

"What the fuck are you on about?"

"I dunno," I shrug, unsuspectingly influenced by the fact that I had been reading psychology books all day yesterday in the library because it had been raining.

"Anyway, me last bird used to complain that I came too early while she had only started to get going. 'How would you like to have sex without coming every time?' she asked me.

I conceded she had a point there. So they next time I fucked her I thought unsexy thoughts: I imagined I was fucking Bernard Manning, but I found that strangely arousing. So I dreamed of Barbara Cartland instead. Mission accomplished! When I felt my woman coming, I let go too. But me bird was still complaining! This time she moaned, 'What, I don't turn you on any more? You don't fancy me enough to prematurely ejaculate!' God, there is no pleasing some women."

"You talk a lot of shit sometimes,"

"Why, thank you, Jonno,"

He resumed his diatribe, on which subject I wouldn't know; my weak attention was focused on the clouds sliding across the skies. Sometimes my view of the clouds was interrupted by nightmarish images, horrible, horrible things – human faces. Thankfully they didn't come too close. Actually, people ambling on the path passing our bench would deviate substantially from their route when they approached us; they would rather get their shoes muddy than be in close proximity to us. They either look down on us or try their best not to look at all. Usually they don't say anything, but when they do I either ignore them or chase them across the churchyard swearing that I'm going to chew their goolies off like any good philosopher would.

The general public look upon us with gargoyle expressions of fear, disgust and contempt. I used to get hurt by it, but the consumption of more alcohol wrapped me up in its inebriate cotton wool and did its job. I mean, what do I care about what other people think of me? Unfortunately I do care. Oh, the joys of being human.

It's nice people feel superior when they see us. People need to feel superior when they are a slave to their jobs, their next pay packet, their HP instalment, and their haemorrhoids. Sitting there, watching people go to work and go about their daily lives, I'm learning something. What I'm learning, I'm not sure exactly. Whatever it is, it ensures that I'll always be on the bench observing it rather than participating in it.

I observe people like a train-spotter spots trains. They all look the same but they have their own numbers and little ineffectual journeys going up and down the same line. But watching people isn't very interesting; it gets boring after a while. One thing I'm certain of is that people are under the mistaken impression that they are special and extraordinary. I am under no such allusions. It is a painful truth. Life throws them at you like pins to a voodoo doll and then expects your subservience to be a happy one. I was never a happy bastard to begin with so I took the path of least resistance, which is conveniently dotted with bars and off licences.

Sometimes, though, I get all self-righteous and say I have had enough of living the loser's script. I tell myself that I am going to go from being an unemployable, law-breaking, alcoholic wanker to being an employed, law-abiding, self-respecting wanker. But when I realise that means having to get off this bench to take a piss, I think, ah, forget it. And besides, I'm just not that evil.

I'm not saying we're not annoying or smelly, but I think the reason we turn people's stomachs is that our uselessness and depravity is on show, explicit, not evil enough to be soberly and constantly held in check. And sitting on a park bench, not working, drinking and swearing, is the full extent of my evil. My evil is just not that evil, my dark side is just not that dark. There's no pretence of defence about our sins, which scares the sobers, and elicits jealousy. Because they have to stay sober. As alcohol obviously disinhibits, they are scared of losing control, they are petrified of showing their true selves. Behind their one thousand masks of convention and self-control, there's an evil clown wanting to make pain to laugh at – the human condition is full of strange lusts. What's the worst part of your soul? A predilection for boy scouts? An appreciation for universal tyranny and the extermination of AIDS sufferers? Auto-erotica in your mother's dress? Forget compassion and decency, apathy saves, apathy immobilises, stops a million sins and crimes in its tracks. I have a mundane lust for apathy. I hold the position of having no position. Because having a position means having to defend it, and I can't be bothered; it means taking time and energy away from drinking and rotting not so quietly, and wasting my beautiful life.

Shithead picked up a discarded paper and we scanned through it. Murmurs of disgust and criticism dribbled out of Shit's mouth. All human beings seem to retain some peculiar arrogance; it's as if you don't feel superior to something or somebody you might as well kill yourself as there doesn't seem to be any point in living otherwise. Drunks are no better. In fact, drunks are the worst offenders. They can have two day old shit in their pants, but they think they have the answers to the world's problems. Not me, I'd rather give problems to the world's answers.

I ignored his words; he wasn't saying anything new. I simply sat there, gulping down my whiskey, waiting for a human to pass by so I could insult them. My luck was in. A whole flood of church-goers were heading our way. Our bench was strategically placed on the only accessible route between the church and the car park, which was another great thing about our bench. I spat into my palms and gleefully rubbed my hands.

I waited for the most pious-looking old bag to pass me by. Of course, she looked down her nose at me. "Awright, gorgeous," I called out to her, "I wouldn't mind   smelling   your   cunt."

The old bag huffed, her face bloated with purple scorn. "Well, really," she sneered, "people like you should be exterminated like vermin."

Well, what a nice Christian attitude she had. Who does she and her cronies think they are? Some Sundays there are more drunks and winos on church property than church-goers. That says a lot about life. The drunks who congregate in the local churchyard are not there for the services, but for something infinitely more religious and holy. In their booze they find God every time, and the dead in the graveyard leave them alone. And, of course, the dead are even greater philosophers than the drunks. I ask the dead questions all the time – and they always give me the same answer:………..

They really know what they are saying.

Out of nowhere Shithead got up and began banging his head against a nearby tree. Shithead used to be a happy, loving, joyful child once upon a time. What happened to him? What happened to me? What has bought him to this point? How did he turn out like this? What and who is responsible? His ordinary parents and ordinary time, most likely.

"Shithead, what are you doing? Stop that!"

He stopped, and turned his head to look at me. "Wittgenstein said," said Shithead, "If you have a pre-recorded universe in which everything is pre-recorded, the only thing not pre-recorded is the pre-recordings themselves."

Shithead then dropped down dead. I cried for him and then called an ambulance, but not before I took all his money and drank all of his booze, of course.

WITHOUT A DRINK

I'm a sober nobody
who politely and quietly lets
the whole world crush me
Give me a drink however
and I'll protest very loudly
and tell all the nice people
of this beautiful world to
"Eff off and leave me the
hell alone."
Without a drink I'm a whore
nobody wants to fuck
but with a glass in my hand
I'm suddenly irresistible and
people can't stop fucking me over.
Without a drink I'm a person
who bloody needs one
Without a drink my conversation
is boring and vapid
lubricated with liquor, however,
I become the world's greatest
philosopher.
Without a drink
life is too painful
and I want to die.
With a drink
life is still painful
But at least I am dying…
… Cheers.

LITTLE LOVE NOTE

I want to kill you
but I won't.
I will just spend
the rest of my life
hating you
with love in my heart.

IT COULD BE YOU

"Shitty fucking Christ. I don't believe this. What a bitch of a day." These curses emanated from the 22nd car stuck in a 200-car tailback on a humid Saturday night. Not only had Mac been stuck in traffic for over an hour, the hot weather was driving him crazy too. In the sickly sauna of his own skin, he was sweating like a monkey in a microwave. His day, up to that point, had been a day of average bad shite, but being stuck in a hot, sticky traffic jam disturbed the flushing mechanism of his toilet equilibrium, thereby paying the fare to set the carousel of his twisted mind in motion again. The longer he spent fixed in this putrid metal standstill, the madder he got. At one point he wanted to blow away every happy-go-lucky human being he saw. But, one: he didn't have a gun; and two: the people on the street outside were too cute for their own good. He also realised that he would merely be displacing his aggression onto innocent parties; he knew the grotesque fountainhead of his rage was himself. Reflecting upon his life always inflamed his soul. He didn't like the feeling, the presence of the soul in this day and age.

What am I doing? What the fuck am I doing? Why am I in a job I hate? Why am I going home to a wife that can't stand me any more? Why am I going home to children who resent me? Right now my wife will be watching one of those Saturday night game shows she loves so much. For a moment Mac was glad he was stuck in endless traffic and not sitting to his wife right now. Dazzled by the sparkling false-teethed smug smiles of game show hosts, his wife would turn to him and say, "Why can't everybody be happy like game show hosts?

Why can't everybody have a smile ready for the world? Why don't you ever smile, Mac? You look handsome when you smile. I don't see you smile any more. Smile for me, Mac, please." Mac felt nauseous with his wife's request. His lips quivered uneasily before forming into a stiff smile. When his wife returned her attention to the game show on the telly, Mac dropped his smile like a lead weight and began privately entertaining thoughts of slitting the game show host's throat slowly. The smile forming on his lips wasn't so fake this time.

Another thing he had to look forward to when he got home tonight – if he ever got out of this traffic jam, that is – were more bills in the post. Plus maybe a letter or two from family members. I prefer the bills to another bloody boring letter from my mother, he sniggered to himself. Bills ask less of my soul. But he knew he was in no position to insult his mother's insipid letters of tedious wisdom. The story of his life would make boring reading too. I'm a futile and insignificant person. We are all futile and insignificant persons.

But you'd better keep hold of your sanity and that smile on your face. If you can't or don't want to take the humiliation or the loss of personal control society promises you, you're weak, inadequate. Be stronger so we can squeeze more blood out of the stone, more mileage out of you on a mediocre road going nowhere. Mac stared down the road that was going nowhere and studied the faces of other drivers: everybody looked pissed off and tense and angry; everybody was probably listening to the news on the radio right now, insulting the politicians mentioned, and cursing the injustices and tragedies of the world. Nobody really likes to adhere to rules and laws of society they think are absurd, venal and facetious, but they do it because that selfsame society provides them with the material things their little greedy hearts desire. Cars, CD systems, etc, are perfect distractions from confronting and dealing with the injustices of the world, or from asking the big questions. Example: life isn't fair, it's corrupt; those in power abuse that power blatantly; there's too much pain, etc, etc. But buying big cars and wide screen TVs ensures we keep the process going, the greedy fed, the feeble multitudes satisfied. The unscrupulous of this world don't take advantage of us, they give us what we want. We are fooled into spending obscene amounts of cash on a car with power-steering, 16 valve engine, and so on, so we can be forever stuck in traffic like this. "BUY. BUY. BUY, MOTHERFUCKER, BUY." It's in your face, it's shoved down your throat like sweetened vomit, it's everywhere – on billboards, shop windows, plastered on the sides of buses, or even on people themselves, or in the hopeful hopeless dreams behind the dead eyes of contemplating pedestrians looking for reasons to be.

One particular ad caught Mac's eye. It was the lottery ad. Here's the perfect example of what I'm talking about, thought Mac. A lot of people oppose and mistrust how the lottery charity funds are awarded; that opera houses get millions and deprived areas get nothing. But we still go out and buy more lottery tickets, turned into hypocrites through desperation. The sign says: 'IT COULD BE YOU'. And everybody's thinking, "It should be me, my pain is greater, my need is greater. I should win. I deserve it. And when you don't win you feel like you've been fucked over.

"After the break we have those lottery numbers coming up for you folks. Stay tuned!" The radio D.J. beamed insincerely.

Mac stayed tuned. He felt his jacket pocket for his lottery ticket; it was still there. Despite himself, Mac began to fantasise about what he'd do with the money if he won. I'd buy my kids everything they ever wished for. Maybe then they'll speak to me nicely. I'd buy my wife all the clothes she wants. Maybe then we'll love each other again. I'll buy a big mansion; it'll give us more freedom (or is it a bigger cage…).

"Here are the lottery numbers folks…" Mac fumbled for his lottery ticket and held it between his thumb and forefinger with a slight anticipatory tremor in his hand.

"The first number is 39…"

Yes, yes! I've got that.

"Next comes number 23…"

Phew, got that too!"

"41 is the next ball…"

Yes, yes. Life is beautiful. The world is as it should be. No need to get worked up over nothing. Every person is beautiful…

"The fourth ball is number 12…"

Mac felt as if he was punched in the stomach; he didn't have number 12. No matter, he told himself, I can still get five numbers and win a decent amount.

"Number 5 is next."

Number 5 was not next for Mac.

"The final number is 2…"

Mac stared at his ticket that took him halfway to heaven then dropped him from the sky without a parachute.

The traffic started moving again. But Mac did not drive home but straight into the river a few hundred metres down the road.

His suicide note was the lottery ticket pinned to his lapel.

LIFE – CHEAP AT TWICE THE PRICE

I don't know what I'm doing
or thinking any more
But then again I'm merely an incompetent
messenger in the house of pain
that is my mind: the rent is ridiculous,
but then the cheapest lives are always
The most expensive to keep.

In my darkest moments
I always see a light somewhere
something to draw me away from death.
So I apprehensively – but hopefully –
approach that light
Only to find it's somebody's death pyre,
or an illuminated sign trying to sell me
something I don't want
at an inflated price

But I have to buy it
because life is precious
and I wouldn't want to waste it now,
would I?

A DAY AT THE SEASIDE

The automatic exit doors of an anonymous seaside town railway station slide open. A man selling inflated balloons stands outside.

"Buy a balloon, luv. It'll brighten up your day. I only have a few left."

The woman who has just left the railway station shakes her head and says, "No, thank you,"

"Come on, they're for charity, for the local children's hospital."

"Okay, I'll buy one,"

The transaction takes place. The balloon seller hands her a balloon with a smiling face printed on it. "There you are, luv, one with a happy face to cheer you up. You look like you need it."

Balloon in hand, the woman walks towards the taxi rank. A cab driver sitting on the bonnet of his taxi jumps up and cheerfully greets the woman. "Want a cab?"

"Er, yes,"

"Where to?"

"The ocean, please,"

"Righto,"

Inside the taxi cab: "It's straight off to the beach for you, then?" the driver asks cordially, "Not going to book into a hotel first? Just here for the day trip?"

"Yes, I'm just here for the day," she replies unemotionally.

"Alone?"

"Yes, alone."

"No boyfriend?"

"No… not any more."

"Oh, I'm sorry about that. But there's plenty more fish in the sea… Plan to go anywhere apart from the beach?"

"No. The ocean's enough for me."

"Going for a swim?"

"You could say that."

The rest of the cab ride is silent. The smiling balloon bounces inanely about inside the cab.

The woman finds a spot on the beach and sits down. She watches the waves roll in and the waves roll out again. Seagulls devour the washed-up fish on the beach.

The woman takes off her shoes and walks down to the ocean; at the water's edge she stops. She ties the string attached to the balloon around her wrist, and walks into the ocean. A few minutes later the woman is face down in the water, dead. The smiling balloon attached to her wrist blows about in the wind.

NO LAUGHTER

No laughter for the divinity of dead clowns
Give death threats to blue skies,
name withheld, of course,
watch repeating oceans of empty mirrors,
where each sunrise has become an idyllic
defamation of the soul.
So return to your games in the playing
ground of eternal loss, while you
microwave your VD dinner
of happy uselessness.
Start what you have finished
Zero times me times the world minus
you
means nothing to me.
I'm dying to live
I'm dying to live
Start what you have finished.

SUICIDE NOTE

I just want to say…
Shit! I don't know what to say.
Life is beautiful?
I'm only killing myself
because I'm a coward?
I look out the window
and I have nothing but admiration
for those of you who have chosen
life: you look a happy, contented
bunch. Fuck, if I have to explain,
you can never know. But you do know…
… don't you?

"Come on, Jo, are you sure you don't want to go to the coast with us. It's your last chance. The car is ready to go."

"Yes, I'm sure."

"We'll stop off at a Happy Eater for lunch."

Jo shrivelled her face in disgust. "Happy Eater, huh, Happy Bulimic, more like. The Happy Eater logo has its finger down its throat, does it not? I'm not surprised, what with all that cheap, synthetic offal they serve up as food. Now I'm definitely sure I don't want to go on your trip. Besides, there's a culinary programme on TV I want to see, one that shows you what real food is."

Danielle looked at her flatmate with a sense of despair. She knew Jo would refuse to come, but she felt she had to ask. She was worried about her friend; Jo's behaviour was becoming more bizarre, reclusive and unhealthy by the day. A trip to the seaside would have done her good, get her out of her shell a bit more. Danielle had known Jo since primary school and they had been best of friends since they were 7, they did everything together. That was until a year ago. Since then, slowly but surely, Jo became more and more withdrawn, keeping herself locked in her room; when she was in the company of others, she was sullen and uncommunicative. Since losing her job, Jo spent the majority of the time furtively watching videos behind the locked door of her bedroom. Danielle was intrigued as to the contents of these secret videos. She envisioned them to be blue movies. On one of the rare days Jo went out, Danielle managed to unlock the cupboard the videos were in and slipped one into a VCR. She was disappointed to see they were nothing more than recordings of operations of various hospital documentaries. Shit, thought Danielle, why all the secrecy in watching these videos if they are not pornographic, if they are not something to be hidden?

Apart from developing strange habits, another odd dimension of her friend's new character was her sudden accident-proneness. Over the course of a few months, Jo had lost four fingers in odd circumstances. What was even stranger the accident-proneness would only manifest itself when Jo was alone. But the strangest thing of all about her accidents in the kitchen was her attitude when the paramedics arrived on the scene. She was indignant that they had been called in the first place, and the paramedics were unable to find her severed digits. Jo's explanation stunned everyone "Oh, I fed them to the dog – he looked hungry."

Jo's psychological state has definitely deteriorated, decided Danielle privately. Though paradoxically she had never seen her friend so physically fit. Jo was obsessed in keeping her body in top condition; she worked out for hours at a time. Why she was so beset in having the perfect body, Danielle had no idea. It wasn't vanity – Jo didn't flaunt her body. And it wasn't to make her more attractive to men – Jo had totally lost interest in the opposite sex. She had lost interest in humanity altogether. And she didn't keep fit for health reasons. Jo let it be known to all that she hated life and wouldn't want to live long. The only conversation people could get out of her was her caustic, bitter observations about the utter meaningless of life.

Danielle let out a sigh of resignation. She cursorily scanned the TV page of the newspaper to see what cookery programme Jo wanted to watch. "Eh?" she mouthed in puzzlement; there were no cookery programmes advertised for today whatsoever. There were the usual repeats and yet another hospital documentary. Danielle shrugged this incongruity off and left the flat to hit the road to the coast. She said goodbye to Jo; Jo stared at her old friend blankly. However, a smile formed on her face when Danielle shut the front door behind her.

Jo switched on the TV. She turned to the channel the medical documentary was on. She licked her lips as the surgeon made an incision on some poor fool's abdomen. It was at times like these Jo missed her job. She felt a slight twinge of regret.

Even though Jo had performed her duties as theatre nurse satisfactorily, the people at the hospital were glad to see the back of her. Why they did not like her was hard to pinpoint really. There was something about her demeanour that was unsettling; it was hard being in the same room as her without feeling very uncomfortable. Something about the way she looked at you, surveyed your body, seemingly with one of the deadly sins consuming her intimidating gaze. It wasn't lust exactly. Envy? No. Gluttony? Maybe…

She was also seen as untrustworthy by the hospital. She developed a reputation as being the hospital kleptomaniac. Whenever she worked in a specific hospital department, things would invariably go missing – bandages, scalpels, sutre sets, clamps, crutches, amputation saws, anaesthetic drugs. One time, en route to a transplant operation, she lost the donated organ entrusted in her keep. The oddest thing to go missing in her care were parts of research cadavers. Suspecting her of selling these spare parts to unscrupulous research laboratories, the hospital searched her bag as she left work one day, after an arm of a cadaver went missing. They found no arm in her bag or on her person. They eventually found the arm – minus its flesh, skin and sinew – stuck in a U-bend. Somebody had tried to flush it down the toilet. To avoid a scandal, and without evidence, they were reluctant to sack her for impropriety. She took her eventual dismissal for health reasons in her stride. She did love her work, but she could hardly keep her mind on the job. Whenever she assisted in intrusive surgery, it was too much for her. It was like an over-sexed teenager being the only male on a desert island of willing females... or an anorexic in a cake shop...

Not only was the local hospital her former workplace, but her supermarket, too, which was proving to be inconvenient, as she was feeling a bit peckish now.

Ah, there's no moaning about it now, Jo thought to herself. She didn't want to have to buy her food; she wanted to be totally self-sufficient. Unfortunately, because she lived in a flat, growing her own food was unrealistic. All she was able to grow were tomatoes and herbs on her balcony. Besides, she liked a bit of meat. Because of things like B.S.E. and battery hens, she gave supermarkets and butchers a wide berth. And she knew she didn't have it in her heart to raise and kill her own animals, especially if they looked up at her with pleading eyes when it was time to slaughter them. She was only capable of killing something she hated – and the only animals she hated were human beings.

Now she wasn't working in the hospital any more, she was without a means of adequate food supply, which meant it was highly impractical to eat other humans anyway. However, whenever she saw an occupied hearse trundling off to deposit its load into a hole in the ground, she admonished the waste of good food.

As her misanthropy increased, so did her distaste for consuming the people behind it. The corpses at the hospital were usually disease-ridden slabs of meat. Eating them was like eating infected, dirty offal, not unlike munching upon a cheap, tasteless burger from a fast food store – quality was definitely lacking. And why have a burger when you can have prime steak – her own body was in tip-top condition. It was also kind of like that saying: 'Every man likes the smell of his own fart.' You usually don't think twice about eating your own bogey, but the idea of eating somebody else's disgusts you.

All she had left to eat in the flat were a few shrivelled tomatoes and a few glasses of Bloody Marys in the fridge. Not only Bloody Marys, but bloody Johns, stupid Sarahs, and an irksome Mr Johnson – names suspiciously similar to those on the blood donor register.

She downed a few glasses but still wasn't satisfied. Her over-riding urge to devour herself was growing with every growl of her empty stomach. Maybe it's better to surrender to this impulse to self-cannibalise. What's the alternative? Struggling financially, mentally, emotionally from day to day for the sake of a beautiful life.

The world was tearing her apart, piece by piece, she could definitely feel the world around her slowly and insidiously consume her being. Why can't I have my share of the cake? Jo asked herself with some degree of exasperation and indignation. It was an act of ultimate self-control – to devour yourself before the rest of the world does.

Apart from that, her body was in constant pain anyway. Tests were carried out but no cause was found. "It's all in your head," her G.P. smirked disdainfully, "psychosomatic." Which meant she had to find her own cure: painkillers did not kill the pain; faith-healers did not heal; acupuncture merely made holes. The only way she would not feel pain was if there was no body to feel the pain. Self-mutilation did not go deep enough for Jo. I not merely content to cut the skin on my arm – I want to saw the damn arm off. I want to gorge my eyes out. I want to extract my teeth with a smile on my face. I want to pour my brain into a blender and drink its juices of rank and tainted ineptitude, Jo asserted forcefully. She was finally ready to shed the futile and profitless – yet delicious – cocoon that was her body.

Jo spread out her array of surgical instruments purposefully. She injected herself with a local anaesthetic in the appropriate regions of her body; when it took effect, she made a deep incision into her left arm at her elbow, cutting through connective tissues. Her job gave her the technical skill to perform the intricate amputation of her left arm. After completing the job and sewing herself up, she ground the flesh of her amputated arm through a mincer and made spaghetti Bolognese with the meat, along with tomatoes, herbs, and a packet of spaghetti past its sell-by date lurking forlornly in the back of an extremely bare food cupboard.

She savoured the thought, as her body digested her own body, that her being was being transformed into shit. How appropriate. What a suitable and befitting fate.

Continuing with her self-dismemberment, her right leg was next to come off; she gormandised it from the top of the thigh down, stopping short at her ankles. Feet, yuk, I can't eat my own feet, Jo whined to herself. She could hear her mother say out loud in her head, "You were always a fussy eater."

However, she did stuff her face with her own face, and ate and drank to her heart's content. Actually, she did drink her heart's content. Needless to say, despite the anaesthetic and careful surgical procedures, the pain was too much, and the blood loss too great: her circulation collapsed and she went into shock. Death came quickly. If she hadn't eaten her own lips, there would have been a smile of contentment on her face.

NOTHING ON THE MENU

A dingy, anonymous café:
cups of coffee, sunlight
on the spoons, on worn-down
tables, chairs, on
worn-down people.
The neon flashes
'Hungry?'
in the window

During a quiet period,
The waitress looks out of the window
Fifteen years of waitressing… shit
Fifteen years of tasting grease in everything
Fifteen years of washing endless dirty dishes
Fifteen years of endless dirty old men smiles
Fifteen years of lewd comments, of being leered at
Fifteen years of politely, coldly letting them.
As she got older, it happened less and less
until they finally ignored her.
She didn't know which she preferred

"I want to die, I want to die, I want to die,"
she'd repeat as a mantra – it helped her to
get through the day.
She realised her life to come would be the same
as her life before: no new loves, no new
experiences, no new thoughts, no new
answers to the big questions, like:
What is the meaning of life?
And is it precious?
It must be if it is so expensive to live it.

And the biggest question of them all:
The sign outside states this is Joe's Café
But who the hell is Joe?

A DAY OUT IN THE PARK

The sun shines. The park flowers are blooming majestically – the day couldn't be more perfect. It's Sunday. Quality time. Picnics. Sunbathers. Happy families. Dripping ice cream cones. Dogs energetically chase sticks and balls. Kites contend with the birds for the skies.

An ordinary-looking man leans against a tree stump, watching all this with a smile on his face. It's the perfect setting for him. Life isn't so bad when it's like this. Even the bees landing on his skin don't bother him. A little girl, having picked some flowers, disengages herself from her family strolling along a path to hand him a bunch of daisies. "Here you are, Mister,"

He grins playfully at the little girl. "Why, thank you, sweetheart. They're lovely."

The little girl giggles bashfully and runs back to join her family. She turns around to say goodbye to him. He waves back, pulling a funny face to make her laugh.

The man opens his canvas tool bag and pulls out a ham sandwich. A passing dog takes an interest in the ham. The man tears off a piece of sandwich and tosses it into the waiting jaws of the hopeful canine, slobbering with anticipation. The dog totters off with a wag in its tail.

A few beautiful women pass him by. He smiles at them. Sometimes he gets a smile back. He delves into his tool bag and pulls out the last item in it. He rises to his feet.

He smiles once again. The machine gun in his hand massacres seventeen people in the park in less than half a minute.

The beautiful sun in the skies stays beautiful.

TAKE IT IN YOUR STRIDE

I do a lot of walking, journeys without destinations,
all the places I pass are mere way stations
to our beautiful eventual nothingness.
On one of these walks I witnessed an armed robbery:
  A security guard got shot in the face; he died instantly
That's funny, I thought. I don't mean funny
as in ha, ha – nobody was laughing.
I thought it was funny that only a few minutes before
the security guard was thinking his boring, ordinary
thoughts, and worrying about his bills, and
pondering what to watch on TV that night.
In all likelihood he wasn't a happy man, and to
top it all off, his starchy uniform was chaffing
him raw on this hot summery day. It's funny
that one moment he was feeling like hell, and then
-    BANG! – he was dead, wiped clean
from existence, extinguished.
At that precise moment his wife was probably
watching a daytime game show; she has no idea
he's dead now. That's strange, very strange indeed.
Then I was hit by a horrible thought:
An awful, anonymous life is better than no
life at all – that's the tragedy.
But his kids will still cry for him
and miss him very much.
I walk away and try not to think about it.
But I do.

NATURAL

I love nature
She's a beautiful goddess
and evil bitch, all rolled
into one sun, one moon,
one earth.
She constantly screams,
"There's too many bloody people!"
So as a form of population control,
she gives us the gifts of disease,
famine, drought, hurricanes,
earthquakes and fire.
But still she screams,
"There's too many bloody people!
And they are chewing on my brain
like maggots!"
We've turned nature into a brain-dead
homicidal
cosmic
non-entity.
But still the sun shines.

LOVE'S FINAL NOTICE

The sunlight slowly washed over the ground I found myself sleeping on. My body was stiff from sleeping on alleyway concrete, and my palate still retained the flavour of last night's nausea. I wasn't sick this morning, though – not physically anyway. Yesterday had been my job interview. I hate job interviews more than I hate doing the actual job. It means coming up with disgustingly happy reasons why you want to surrender your soul to some form of spurious, bland servility. I can't do it without either wanting to kill myself or piss myself with laughter. Yesterday was no exception. Midway through telling a personnel manager why it was my ambition to work in a toilet roll factory, I stopped reading from the bad script of the bad play society had concocted, and vomited all over his desk. The faltering interview was effectively over at that moment. Without even bothering to apologise, I just got up and left.

Now the D.S.S. would be stopping my dole money for sure. Puking over the personnel manager's desk was worse than not turning up for the interview. But I no longer cared. I had enough money in my pocket to get drunk and 1001 ways to commit suicide in this fair city. So last night I got drunk – but ended up too tired and sick to kill myself.

My agenda for today was to consume vast amounts of alcohol for breakfast, and then commit anonymous suicide for lunch. I sat up and examined myself. I still had my life, still had money in my pocket, and I still had my knickers on. So it was obvious I hadn't been murdered, robbed or raped during my alleyway sleep. Humanity was evidently in a benevolent mood last night.

Or maybe they just couldn't find me – the alleyway was a good hiding place. I got up onto my unsteady feet and, with my hangover guiding my steps, I made my way to a public convenience.

At a public convenience sink I washed myself as best as I could. The taste in my mouth was ugly. So I gargled with water and chewed my last stick of chewing gum to freshen up my breath. Then I washed myself with warm water and sticky dispenser soap. It was at this point I got into an argument with the lavatory attendant. She told me I wasn't allowed to wash myself at the sink – it was only for hands. "Where am I supposed to wash, then – in the toilet?" I retorted. "Why is it your problem? I'm not going to leave a mess behind. You won't even know I've been here." This was a blatant and obvious lie. But I couldn't placate the old cow. She seemed to be drowning in a permanent black mood. But then wouldn't you be the same if you worked for less than the recommended minimum wage and had to clean after people unable to shit into the actual toilet. I felt bad. So apologised, cleared up, and left.

Once outside, I got rid of my coat. It was dirty and advertised too many of last night's deadly sins, such as sloth, lust and gluttony. The morning was chilly, but my long walk to Soho, where I knew some illegal all-night bars operated, would warm me up.

I sat myself at the end of the bar. It was on top of a sex shop, so there were the obligatory dirty old men drinking upstairs as well. If the porno mags downstairs couldn't lift their, erm, souls, overpriced alcohol would. A few tried to hit on me – they thought I was some over-sexed housewife. And, of course, they were right. But I wasn't interested in thirty second intercourse. Why fucking bother? I'd get more passion, love and attention out of a vibrator.

But their hard-ons soon changed directions. Another woman entered the bar. I couldn't blame them – she was absolutely beautiful. Don't make me describe her physical attributes here on the page, I won't be able to take it. Two fucking days after splitting up with her, I am trying to write objectively the story of how we met, after three acrimonious years together. Our love finally became ugly, hurtful, so what's the use of bringing beauty into the story. The gun next to this computer doesn't need any more excuses to be used.

Back to the story however…

Despite their hard-ons and fat butts, the men in the bar suddenly found room next to themselves for her to sit.

But she sat next to me.

When it was obvious they were going to have more luck with the rubber dolls downstairs, the male clientele of the bar soon left to return to their unhappy jobs and even unhappier wives.

The summer sun hadn't totally eradicated the unsunned ring mark of her wedding finger. I spotted this as I indulgently savoured her being as she drained drink after drink.

"You want another drink?" I finally had the courage to ask her.

"That's a stupid question, isn't it?"

"I guess it is," I ordered more drinks for myself and Sara. "Just got divorced, huh?" I always say the wrong things, ask the wrong questions. My conversational skills aren't well developed. But then again I've never had anything worth saying.

Sara rubbed the pale shadow of her discarded ring. "Yes, I've just got divorced. What about you – are you married?"

"No, I've never been married. Been divorced plenty of times, though."

"Eh? Well, my husband, I mean my ex-husband wanted me to stop drinking and become a dutiful wife."

"So you divorced on the grounds of mental cruelty?"

"You could say that. He said my drinking was driving us apart. I had to disagree with him – it was what kept us together."

"Why's that, then?"

"There's one thing I'm grateful to my alcoholism for."

"What's that, then?"

"Heterosexuality."

So that was how we met. After, we went to her flat to make love. I postponed my suicide. I decided to take the slow way out – love.

Why am I writing about how we met now that we are no longer together? Because the best suicide notes are love stories – and vice versa. Well, this first chapter will be the last. I can't go on any more – with life or this fucking story.

So here is the final chapter.

BROKEN

A dripping tap can drive U insane
Like your own heart beating to
a rhythm you can't adjust to.
Yes, my heart is a faucet
losing itself drop by drop, silently
in its own corner
Just making enough noise
to annoy whoever is listening.
Drip – a liquid discard of soul in instalments
Drop – all day
Drip – every day.

STREET SATORI

Pausing in my step
I saw something beautiful
The people who shared
the pavement with me hated
my existence in an instant
without even knowing me
cursing me for slowing down
their great, important
worthy journeys. I stepped
aside and let them go
Let them be with their own
coveted uselessness.
I looked down, by my feet:
The sun was shining
into a puddle,
and raindrops were giving me
a thousand variations of
Cosmic beauty.
Was I the only person to see it?
Why is that?
Because it doesn't pay the bills,
so let's chuck it out.
I'm glad I look through other
people's rubbish then.

ELEVATION

"You know how to press my buttons," he snarled.
"Why don't you press mine," I told him. "I have
a million floors of self-loathing, disgust, love
and sunshine… Jump from any story you want.
I've got loads of them too.
You're stuck between floors
Stuck in the lift with me, and the piss and shit
of those before us.
There's nothing to do but screw our brains out
and wait for elevation."

PROZAC WHORE

I'm a Prozac whore
An existence bore
A rotting fruit of knowledge core
The perfect flaw
The dead bird soar
But mostly I'm a Prozac whore
I'm chemically delirious
I'm so happy I could take
the whole bottle
Suicide is a toilet
I won't flush
Death is a thing I won't rush
Tattoo smiley faces
on my scars
Show the world that I'm
Happy, trigger happy
Let me fulfil my agenda
of inconsequence
Living for every new day
that comes
ejaculating prematurely
into the void
I love the sun
but hate the day it brings
like a bad aftertaste
So sun
I will rise high enough
To shoot you down
One day
One day.

EATEN MIRROR

I seem to monopolise the psychic bureaucracy of
stupidity
So douse my pain in bleach
Drown my laughter with gasoline
My eyes take pictures I wish I could tear up
Life is a two-dimensional pain, an
eaten mirror where snakes swim in my brain
I'm going to commit suicide on my birthday
It's the best present life has ever given me
When I go to hell, I'll say hi to the devil for you

GOD'S SUICIDE NOTE

I'm God
I hate my fucking job
Do you want it?
Even the devil wouldn't have me
I created billions of minions
to bow down before me
But not one will suck my dick
except this leery witch called Mary,
who wants child support
payments for eternity,
the bitch.

I said do not eat from the tree
of knowledge. I wanted humans
to be dumb sacks of shit. It
made me feel good or something.

I remember one angelic fucker
took me, God, hostage.
He sodomised me, the bastard,
and then he said, "You created
everything here, God."

So on the eighth day, God surveyed
everything around him and said,
"What the hell have I done?… Shit…
Goodbye cruel world…"
And committed suicide.

It was heavenly.

WRITE YOUR OWN SUICIDE NOTE HERE:

THEN PUT IT IN THE FUCKING BIN

THE MAENAD ANGEL POETICS

By

DOLLY SEN

Published by:
Chipmukapublishing
PO Box 6872
Brentwood
Essex
CM13 1ZT
United Kingdom

www.chipmunkapublishing.com

DOLLY SEN BIOG

Dolly Sen was born on 23rd October 1970 in London,
where she still lives.

"I had my first psychotic experience aged 14 and
stopped going to school. A series of dead end jobs
followed. Pretty early on I decided I didn't want any
more of the 9-5 shit and spoon race, and began to
write… and maybe watch 70s cop shows."

Dolly Sen is a writer, director, artist, film-maker, poet,
performer, raconteur, playwright, mental health
consultant, music-maker and public speaker. Since her
much-acclaimed book 'The World is Full of Laughter'
was published by Chipmunka in 2002, she has had 3
further books published, had a succession of
performance roles around Europe and places like The
Young Vic, Trafalgar Square and The Royal Festival
Hall; did a poetry tour and won a poetry award from
Andrew Motion; directed two plays and several films,
appeared on TV, and has done spoken word at City Hall
and Oxford University.

This is staggering since she dropped out of school at 14
and has no formal qualifications. She has also had to
share her life with severe mental health problems. She
was told she would never amount to anything but would
end up in jail or Broadmoor and she believed this and

was on her way there when she changed her belief into the one of believing she could do anything she wanted to do.

This proves that the mind is an amazing thing; it can drive you mad and inspire you in the same breath. And that you can do anything if you believe you can do it.

This I say:
You burn
urban decay
Soulless replay
Of a life in front of the TV
Giving cerebral VD
TV is your teacher
Your preacher
Your prosthetic lecher
No sublimation
Just alienation

I'm an angel no one
Wants the help of
I'm the angel of the truth
nobody wants to hear
Nobody listens to my story
Of spiritual outlawry
Every time I tell it
I'm taken to a place of safety
Where my soul is ripped in sections

Stripped of my keys, I cannot sing like an angel
Stripped of my keys, I don't have a home
Stripped of my keys, I am in a cell

They call me the bag lady
But I need the bags to carry my wings

The beautiful tyranny of my own inconsequence

The womb where I came from

Smoked a pack a day
Cried lonely in a bedsit
My father has finally forgiven
Me for my birth

We're not gods or super humans
We are people in our own cells
And viscera
In a bag of skin
With a brainwashed brain
Being brainwashed
By other washed brains

I have the talent of turning
People dysfunctional in a minute

Soul death while U wait

Why not go mad, eh?

We're happily living in
Mediocrity
Where dignity and integrity
Are abnormal,
Feared traits in a human being.

Give the rat race rat head
Your big mouth on the small dick
Of the 9-5 ogre

Prisms of dead colours
Shine
In a heart turned

Inside out

Pain in the trees
I see pain in the trees
The skies are blue about it
And the clouds go by without
Even looking down
Unable to carry the weight
Of its own tears

The indigo sunset
Turns its back

Giggles of small children
Grow up,
And die

I have to kill my father
To make him a better human being
An imploding star
In my celestial remorse

I've got the heart of a dog
Chasing its own tail

I rage at the stage
Where we all perform detestable
Dramas for the entertainment
Of blind gods
Which lead to happy slaves
And even happier graves
The closing down sale of my soul
Everything must go

All bankrupt stock
Now available in black and blue

I want to turn my pain
Into a morgue

It's hard to see the ones you love die
It's even harder to see the ones you hate live

"The only time I'll be happy
to see you is when you're six
feet under."
Parents say the nicest things.

I smiled and loved and laughed
As a child
Growing
Growing
Growing
Gone
I found my place in the world
-     the madhouse

An empty room
A ticking clock
Measuring your eternal absence
With the vanity of the second
Taking all the time in the world
Oblivion is not total
I am aware of it.

Everyone's an angel
Your sanity calls that madness

Your sanity's
Your vanity
There's no room in the mirror for you
Your mirror is on backward

Earthquake
Heartbreak
Somewhere
Something
Breaks

The sweetest thing
Decays
Hardness
Burns your teeth
And swims in your bones

The filth and the folly
Of metronomic
Holy
Holy
Solely

'Step into the light'
poltergeist
zeitgeist

I'll make you rave to the grave
What is it your dancing to?

I'm waiting for Godot and the 59 bus

All couch potatoes
Are ghouls of nato
Your disgust into inaction
Helps their moral misconstruction

All winos on benches
Are philosophers
'Locke, I Kant give a flying Spinoza!'

South London streets
Are not paved with gold
But with used condoms
Of angry, transient lusts
And paid cunts
That look more like scared
Young girls to me
Who've never had a hug.

Where's the soul
On the dole?
Where's the life
In the 9 to 5?
Life's full of choices
But where is my voice
In all this?

Why doesn't God pay my rent?

The skies are godless, thank fuck
They belong to the birds and sun
That's holy enough for me.

Totalitarian eggcups

In Judas symmetries
The loneliness of the sun
That keeps us alive

Or Halparadol Babylon
The sea will always be
Bigger than its own aloneness

The aerosol seer
Gives a breath of fresh air
With consequence
And holes in the argument

In this world of mirrors
People turn their backs on you

To think the day after I die
The sun will rise again
Someone will fart
Someone will cry
Someone will pull a trigger at their own head
All this will go on
Life goes on
It doesn't need me
It doesn't need any of us
It just needs an inside-out flower

One light bulb on all night
Makes me a moth to a flame
Kerosene is my air

I want a higher education
That those in the know

Don't know

Don't bring me back down to earth
I know it's the place of my birth
But it's sad, mad and bad
And I can only make it worse

Cheap life opaque
Gives me empty days

Fuck! This is crazy
Ugly utopia promised me
Carnivals and carousels, turning, turning
Killing
Time. But it's all a hoax
I
Still see
Life
I'm an inmate to the
Fall back down to
Earth. I want the end.

Life is a language ill spoken
Sick of being said

Life ahead
Fate a noose

I'm in my skin
Of aloneness and sin
And full of nothing left

Life is a sick joke

And the punch line
Is death

Ha, ha, ha

But he draws me near
And tells me to taste
The sweet indigo night
With him

Who said suicide is spiritual masturbation?
I bet he was a wanker

The power of love
Has a short fuse
And there's nothing for the meter
And there's nothing for the mile

But his touch makes me lose my skin
Sex on a beach
The ocean our blanket
Our empty shrine
Of squalid nourishment
And sweet corruptions

Drowning into the night
I would be happy
To let the liquid blanket
Warm in perpetual slumber
And blind my vision azure

But as this deadland
Silence

Screams its
Lullaby
We make love
In a world of noise

Air, the thing that keeps us alive
Is nothing
It's nothing

We look at each other
And know blindness can see
Tears decree
A mirror with reflections of you
- even though you've gone.

Close you eyes, baby
See what I'm feeling?
See what I mean?

Close your empty hand
And touch what I feel
Without you
Close your empty hand
And hold me

Close. Close
Yet so far.

I'm ripped to pieces
Noiseless on the velvet decline
Panic. Pain
The adagio wander to the grave

Poisoned by the
Asylum of my dreams begging for
Reality, my mind –crowded inside
And out – tells me there are
No strings attached to the
Opulent noose of existence, that
I am just
A little paranoid

If orgasms are oceans
Then in my being, my body
All the oceans of the earth
Wash under my skin
When you kiss
When you touch
When you fuck
When you love
But why am I standing at the ocean alone now?

The ecstasy
Of you next to me
In a world that likes to
Keep its distance
Forfeit the piracy
Of my ocean
The inadequacy of celibacy
When you smile

Listen to that
It's not silence
But the echoes
Of all the things I couldn't say.

Poetic lesions
Watching incomprehensible seasons
Manic
I can cause global panic
Smile at me and feed my pain
Point a gun to your head
so I can smile again
tell me lies –
so the world has truth again
Do you believe in your ego's
Advertising campaign?
You new and improved recipe
For soul death

It is the maenad's duty
To undertake frenzied writes

To stop following the end point of sanity
Which is the mushroom cloud
I have a sunny disposition

Return me to my nightmares
If this is reality.

What makes a poetic tic tick?

The end point of the road
Leads you back to the beginning
The thing you ran away from
Is the only thing that welcomes you home

How do you like
My vampyric

Soundbites?

Exposed to the sun
My frozen heart decays
Life put it in the freezer
Telling me I would not have any
Use for it

Consigned
science to
The self-reliance
Of it blindness
I prefer kindness

I've got evil all backwards
And my dog too

This is it
I'm in the snake pit
On the ward
With a 100 other gods
The spit
The shit
The piss
The lick
That takes your skin off
The smile
That burns your wings off
The pills
The soul kill
Jack and Jill
Fell down the multinational hill
The milk spills

I cry
I die
I lie
Just to swim out
Of the snake pit
Of burning fish
This is no place of safety
This is where the grave should be
I let Trotsky the pigmy
Sing about envy
I am the ventriloquist dummy
Of the stars.

The sin of skin
The skin of sin
The sin of the sun
And the son of the sin

I need an exorism
Every time I kiss him
Is it a prism
Or a prison?

I'm a hobo 'ho
Ho ho
No no
Let's go
Ride the rail
Impale the failure

Peace together
The mosaic of paranoia
To see the bigger picture

The laughter of the sun
The laughter of the sun
The laughter of the sun

In the desert of humanity
A puddle of thorazine is an oasis

Metal shampoo
For the eye on me
For the iron me
For the irony

Getting drunk on Saturday to unwind
By Sunday morning there's blood on the ground
Your Monday to Friday
Is nothing but let's die day
The 9-5 is a blood sport
What is being hunted exactly?

The taxes of sin are death
Means I have a dodgy syntax

I like peacing together the ice cream
The carousel is making its own flavour
I am ice cream wheels on the sun
Turning inside the burning
Learning inside the yearning
I'm still here.

There is an art to life
Bob Ross

Sex god
Too many gods
And not enough Bods
Bod, what was your road?
I prefer the magic roundabout.

We are all gods
Watching tv
And old dramas

Nobody has any faces any more

Expanded consciousness
On a pin head
Is there a point?

You spin me right round
Baby right round
Like a record
Time
To
your
own
death

facelessness
in the eye scream
dreaming
of a dream
being a dream
that wasn't a dream

life is narcissus anonymous

death can't bear to look in the mirror

the clouds never
touch the streets

broken glass
bare feet

I'm pissing my life away
The urine
Sublime
Of time.

Timeless
Is rhymeless

This is where the crime is

I'm watching butterflies burn
It's your turn

I'm the jester
From Leicester
No, actually I'm from London

I'm really a molester
Of the siesta
In polyester

Oh, the rhyming dictionary is so much fun

The oblivion is nothing but colours

The eyelids no closure

The open all hours
Flowers

I am the pacifist
In love with the gun
The killer
In love with...
someone

the head
tripped
over something

This book is full of
Haiku
Fuck yous
And I love yous

Reality is in the
I
Of the beholder

Which means the world
Is getting colder
And hell
Is a little bit
older

I accept the sun's nepotism in
Allowing the night
To look over me

I see graves,
These bones
That were once
Their parent's
Flirting smile.

I look into eyes
And see they believe
Their parents' lies
I see they've already written
On their graves
'I didn't bother to live'
It's do or die
You could die today
Or are you already dead?
Come on and live
Or have you already made your bed.

Narcissism
Cynicism
Nihilism

I'm an angel
An astral wastrel
My only message is: 'LIVE!'
I shout this on the street
People think I'm crazy

There is no satisfaction in being
An angel
Nobody wants to be saved.
But rather enslaved

Why?
I cry
As pigs take me back
To the sty
I just don't get it
Fed ex the shit

I asked Dali for the time
The mocha tick-tocker

The cellular degeneration
Of
Eternity

I've thrown away the key

They are locking me up
For my own good
Goodness
Is a crime?

The sun is the light
Of a billion minds
That's why it's giving me
Cancer

The special k
Skin
Is in

Death always wins
Yet it doesn't want to
It just waits

To be hated
By everyone
What fun

Time to
Finger fuck
Lady luck

The holy hole
The lonely soul
Those that hold the power
Cannot hold the flower

Heaven is a subsidiary
Of a pharmaceutical company

So I'm on the road
Forever

Coming?

The only baggage I have
Is my wings

Is life
A flight of fancy

The beauty of the breeze
Almost lifts me off my feet

The beauty of the sun
Shows the only number is one

The ocean
The only magic potion

For the pain that is
The rain

My home
My doorway Eden
No food on the tree of
Knowledge

I'm hungry
I'm really hungry
I beg for money
And people spit on me

I try to save their souls
And the police take me away

Have you ever tried LSD
On ECT
God cackles
And demons use your brain
As a comfortable chair

The meaning of life
Is not a sound bite

In case of fire
Break the looking glass

In case of liars
Kiss my arse

The dirty grace
And purity
Of chaos

It's the only thing
The world understands

I'm a trans
Dental
Nurse

So make yourself comfortable
And open wide
Your vacant soul
Needs a filling
It's only going to hurt
A little bit

Forget calories
And salaries
And just live!

∎∎∎

Madness and genius
Are bedfellows
It all depends on who
Is giving who
The head

The head on a platter
The mind over matter

The mad hatter
With the bright eyes
Caught in the headlights
Of a truck

FUCK!

Wittgenstein said: 'If you have a pre-recorded universe
in which everything is pre-recorded, the only thing not
pre-recorded is the pre-recordings themselves'.
But who recorded 'Neighbours'
Over the ending?

All smiles have sadness
Because death will always
Have the last laugh

■■

Are you sure you're not wearing a black triangle?
In Nazi Europe, prostitutes were interned in workcamps
as punishment.
What's the difference between them and the 9-5ers?

Stop being a cog in the sordid machinery of modern
times
Be a particle of a higher planet

Or revert back to being a walking, talking human-skin
lamp
with the light switched off by order of your beautiful,
beautiful life

Work will make you free

Walk under a zyclone sunshine

One of the six million soul holocaust rush hour

Is my soul in the lost property dept of the universe?
staffed by the mundane bureaucracy of the ego?
Watching people rush the hour of their doom so they
can have yet more doom
The perks of the job of being a creature of banal grace –
an
Afterlife?
Please no. We do not need uselessness to proliferate
Into celestial realms.

This is the shape of things to come

Black triangle.

This is the shape of things to come

Black triangle

This

Is

The

Shape

Of

Things

To

Come

In the hope of something better,
you are quite
happy
to do a job you
hate, quite
contented to be a
cog in the machine
just so you can acquire
goods, pay taxes, and go
out every Saturday night,
while you slaver after your
unfulfillable dreams,
because there is nothing else
you can do. You
can look around you – at your
mortaged house, your furniture
bought on credit, at pictures
of your estranged spouse, at
photos of your children
who resent you.
You can look at them
and say these things
are worth it. OR
you can put your hop
around your neck

and walk on air.

Knocking on the door of my own emptiness
Nobody's home
Nobody's left either
Nobody on the other side to open the door but me
I may have to burn down the house
To be let back in
I thought I was on a long journey
But I didn't know it was to back here again
So here I am
Knock, knocking on my own emptiness
Waiting to be let into

Death

What is death but

Silent Laughter now
Fear of the dark is only the darkness now
Trophies glint in junkyards
Children playing
Children playing
– where have they gone?
All the work you did just built a nicer grave
Your loneliness – even lonelier
And your home – the loneliness of all
People – People – Gone – Gone
Where have they gone?
Not here
Not here
Anymore

It's time
To get on the road
To go 'there'.

In my car
leaving everything behind
No more bills or TV
I am going to find myself
if I'm not already forever lost
I'm going somewhere…
anywhere that isn't here
but here is always here
and there is always there.
I've been nowhere special;
the postcards I have sent to myself
have told me that much

But I'm happy, driving alone,
on this empty road.
That's what freedom is…
                              isn't it?

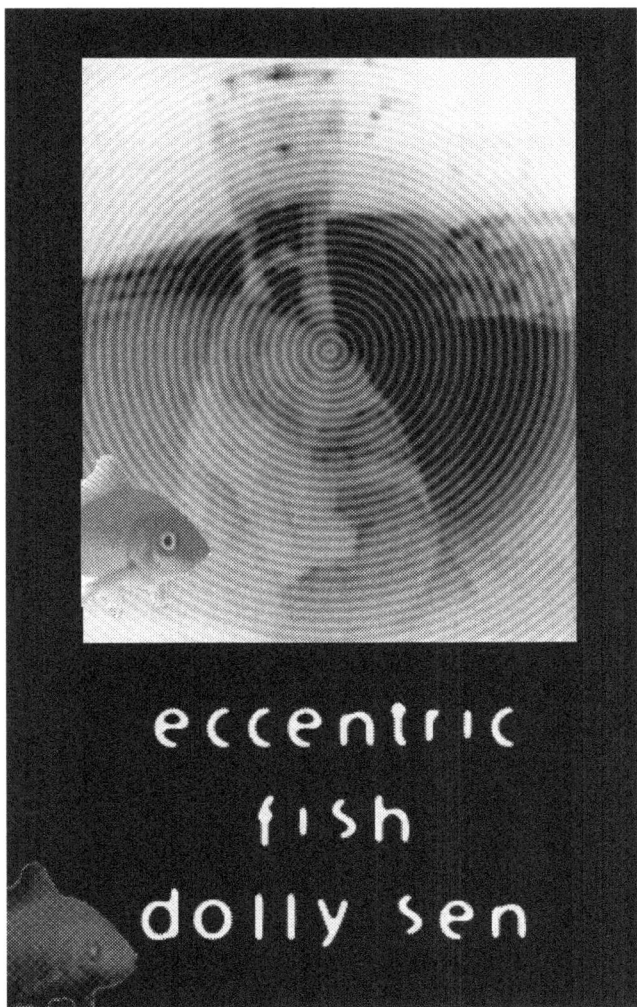

ECCENTRIC FISH

poems by Dolly Sen

Published by:
Chipmukapublishing
PO Box 6872
Brentwood
Essex
CM13 1ZT
United Kingdom

www.chipmunkapublishing.com

dedicated to the memory
of Rachel Rutherford-gill
12 March 1964-17 Nov 2000

Eccentric Fish

Eccentric fish swimming in set concrete
But still making the shore
Still seeing the sun
Still growing flowers
Still smiling in a world of endless liars

Pavement Poem

Do not step here
my dreams have fallen
out of my pocket, and
are hard to find again.
Don't grind them into the ground
Otherwise I will have to wait
for the rain to run into the cracks
to the feed the daisies
to push them back up again.

IS LIFE

Is life the growing of the body
and the hating of the mind,
the shrinking of the soul?
is life being an angel with
amnesia
being an ineffectual demon
stunted by a kind heart
Is love a spanner in the working
of the clouds, tearing them apart
so as to see the sun better,
lips taste tears from the same body
a transparent cannibalism
a rain that
acupunctures to keep the sickness going
that self mutilates with cotton wool

what is this breath about
to sing words into balloons
till they burst?

the big bang drowns
out answer to the meaning of life

but it is pretty to watch.

Is old age the shrinking of the body
and are we still hating the mind?

death drowns out the
answer to life

Nobody is listening anyway.

SPYCHOSIS

let's go fly a kite &
see wombs reject clouds
I've got the hole word in my hand
crucified by candy floss
I throw out the rubbish
and find my dreams
which ones are recyclable, I don't know.

Second-hand slumber is not so bad,
sleeping in your dreams is good enough
Something must be rested
Do you realise you never look in your diary in dreams
you always know what to do next.

Waking is putting on the body again
I never seem to find one that fits.

The smile is cut out to provide a spyhole
my paranoia gets stuck between my teeth

It's a grind.
I am hungry now.
I have fallen down a hole
surviving on catatonic toothpaste
till my rescue.

My silent screams have fresh breath.

Welcome to my dream
there is no admission fee
and you will leave something behind anyway

AND/ORGASM

Head thrown back in ecstasy
to see the stars fall on my face
and travel down the length
of my body
to exit
as
an
electric
flower
Orgasm, a star
that dissolves the skin
turns blood into the speed of sound
The heart sings beautifully
without knowing the words
to the song.
Everything is on a cosmic scale
Bliss creates and destroys worlds in an instant
my nerves orbit an imploded universe
chaos theory as orgasm

Chaos theory as love
is that you and I are here together
in the smiling rain
our eyes seeing only each other
in a world that is collapsing around us...

NOTHING NEW

There is nothing new in dying
There is nothing new in pain
yet it always feels fresh, a flower
that hates itself.
It's just this pain,
this dying
has my name, my face,
but not my permission nor my
understanding
So I play in the field of lost
memories, with a 1000 of my faces
unrecognisable
"I have been here before." the future says.

This is easy to overlook.
stop thinking about what you don't remember
and create forgettable memories
without me

DISTANT BLUE

Skies are distant blue
Beautiful
But there's separation
The scenery in the distance can never be
grasped; it needs you to be far away from it
she doesn't want to be far away from it
She wants to cup the sky
and take it home with her
But always go back empty-handed.

Haikus

My life is my art
every day is a different colour
today is purple

Dog walkers
on a winter common,
a muddy dog is happiness

Jesus is alive
in a padded cell
crucified by bad hospital food

Swans Seeking Liars

Even the sun wants something from me
As the puddles shine my shoes
I toss a coin into a tree
And watch the rain give me change
The chopping block likes to give head, I've found
As I look in the glint of her eye
And the guillotine of her smile
I try to live again guided by
Maps of catatonia and kisses of water
Seeking fires
And endless swans seeking liars

The Window

The sun rose.
She was looking at it angrily, at the window.
The force of her stare only delaying
the sun's ascent for a flash;
her eyes burned.
Tears formed.
But the skies outdid her in that too:
clouds dimmed in the sear of sun,
absorbing the bloodbath of light;
A heart was lost in the process.
Her lover was in bed, in shadow,
her shadow.
She smiled.
I can steal the sun from her at least.

RUNNING OUT

Psychiatrist conference
free pens!
I took one
before I went to talk to docs on
what it is like to be mad
The ink was temperamental:
wrote only half the words
nobody knew what I wanted to say.
I scream in frustration – arrggghh
but those are not my words
just what you made me say
Psychiatrist, read between the lines
stop giving me things that do not work.

This is not a poem but a moan but I put it in the book
anyway.

Choice

Head resting on your belly
Between breast and pussy
I don't know where I want to put my mouth
Inch it higher slowly
Or much, much lower to get lost in you
Choices
Is a journey of tastes
I would rather swallow you whole, leave my skin to
share yours
I have to make do with kisses that draw you soul to yr
skin
And then leave me again
Breath, a deep, deep breath, the mouth rises along the
body
Moving slowly, barely touching, taking you through the
nose,
The mouth, the tongue, the skin.
I write on your skin, the word bliss with my tongue, no
full stops, the sentence trails off........
A mouth that climbs a mountain, meets the sun and a
thousand falling stars
Just to go down again..........

I remember red

I remember red postboxes that no postman collected letters from.
The post office closed it up many times but the metal cover over the mouth of the postbox would never stay on. Stickers and posters
warned the postbox was no longer in use but still people posted their letters.
I said to one of them 'Letters here aren't collected. I mean, look how many letters are stuck in there.'
But the lady still posted her letter.
Who are they writing to? Especially if they know it will never reach their destination.
Letters that had to be written but better left unsaid.

RAZORBLADE WINGS

my angel wings
are made of razors
flight just cuts me to pieces
the more I try
the more you'll find
of me on the floor
clouds self-mutilate
the sun cannot heal
and the winds lie
and the earth believes it
and hides its hurt
in bruised fruit,
shy mountains
and birds that have forgotten the words
to the song.

THE NIGHT IS A TEST

The night is a test.
But it is too dark to see the questions
Let alone the answers
Stars that have already died have asked me to stay
So I stay
They are lonely too
In the knowledge they will be outshone by
Morning every time.
Light always outshines the darkest night
Dawn is suffused by
A light that is orgasmic;
It seduces the air and my mind
Life has become beautiful again.

Water talks
and says, "I am not your tears,"
I am more than that.
an ocean is my swallowed hope,
 you can cry forever
but I will outdo you still

I cannot absolve you
water cannot pull the darkness out of a human heart
even with the razor tapestry of tides
I can stop the heart, but the darkness will shine on
Reflection. Reflection. Reflection.

Water talks, writes on your skin, a bath of catatonia, a
rain of interpolation,
not to be able to finish the sentence
but to give a thousand full stops on your skin
I touch you
The Braille melts
the words wash away.
Take back what you say.

And I am left with water that talks
a foreign language
- I do not know how to listen…

THE LIBEL OF SANITY

I am not an open book. But you can read me in the
Braille of crumbling walls, if anyone bothers to feel, to
feel.

Getting higher
is getting deeper
peel the layers
the colour scheme of dreams

Empty rooms have their lullabies. Empty rooms have
their dreams.

My stream of consciousness is chlorinated, sanitised for
public use, but look under the surface, dive deeper, get
under my skin, come into my dark corners and see how I
judge the world.

I stand because of these walls, but I can never leave
these doors. My head is in the clouds, but I am stuck to
the ground, I would like to weigh myself in mid-flight.
But I am like a bird trying to fly in set concrete.

The libel of sanity. Can you prove reality exists in a
court of law? Where are the witnesses? Where is the
evidence? Except the invented evidence. You build the
walls and say reality exists within these walls? Take the
walls away and what have you got?

The jury is out.

Written from the Heart

Written from the heart
the ink should be blue
but is red

so I lie before anything
has even been said

what should I say?
the heart's lexicon
is not used to coming out of these lips

Put yr head on my breast and listen to my heart
Put yr head on my breast and listen to my heart

Please write my life story
I want to know what happens next.

FLICKER

Dreaming dreams that are at odds with the world,
I open my eyes.
The world brands beauty; the scar is precious,
healing is unkind.
Burning our tears on hidden pyres that sing
with swans and dance

with liars

and tears that meet the stars halfway
just disappear, evaporate
Fire and tears turn into clouds
The rain falls
but we do not know its story.

PLEASE DON'T TOUCH

Spit stains corners the mouth that can't explain
Scars mean some human contact in his life
Detritus on his head, in his head
Grey hand holding that blue can
Inducing disgust in every fucking human that passes
His unwashed absolution ensuring
The distance of everyone
So no-one can see the tears in his eyes

Anger is Eating Clouds for Breakfast

Anger is eating clouds for breakfast, washed down with a little sun that gets stuck in your throat, followed by the picking of teeth with lollipop ladies.

Anger is going clothes shopping, and choosing a skin three sizes too small, and a heart three sizes too big.

Anger is spending the lunch break trying to fit a volcano in a thimble, and losing hope in a bowl of sugar cubes.

Anger goes home, fries snowflakes in the frying pan, and complains there is nothing to eat.

Go to the fridge and find your smile in a milk bottle and pour it over your head anger.

Rain is my Skin

Rain is my skin
You can see right through me
The lies I hide
stain; clouds form,
and truth will not set me free
Break the stained-glass
that is my heart
to be clear:

A storm is heading your way.

"Did you sleep well?"
"No, I made a few mistakes."
Steven Wright, Comedian.

SLEEP WALK

Did you sleep well?
No, I made a few mistakes.
The truth keeps interupting.
I don't know how to end the dream.
I forget to dot the tease
And cross the eyes.
Poor Dali,
Making movies on how I see the world
With dyslexic dogs
Providing the subtitles.
Don't read the small print.

The truth keeps interupting.
I don't know how to end the dream.
I can read the film
Of existence
It is transparent
Dreams are commercial breaks
Selling my soul back to me
But I want more:
33% extra soul
buy one soul, get one free
I want new and improved soul
With a fresher fragrance

So it is hard to sleep well
I am sleep-walking on the hot coals
Of the stars,
One day I will get to the end

And not wake up.

TODAY

Today you are as half as far
But still too distant
I love you
but you do not want to hear
these words
silence flays my skin
I cannot be touched
any more

BINARY CODA

The binary code of the doze
the existential lullabies
sing me lies
sing my pain to sleep
Am I one or am I none?
Am I one or am I none?
Am I one or am I none?
Am I one or am I none?
Am I one or am I none?
Am I one or am I none?

I am none I am none I am none
I am done
with
dreams

I am done with the poetry of freedom

because the only time you hear it nowadays is
in car commercials

the human condition
the burning of flowers under
kerosene as rain

Sometimes none is better than one.

SKIN

Skin on skin is still 2 skins, 2 separate bodies. I want to bury myself in you, my skin disappearing like clouds in the most golden of suns.

Alone, my body can be measured, with you it is infinite. Alone, my skin can be measured. With you, skin is ocean, skin is sky, you are a dream that knows no morning, skin is the insanity and straitjacket both. Skin separates me from you.

But...

Skin is how I touch you too. Skin is dusk, dawn, skin is sun, warmer as it gets closer to me, fire when there is finally connection.

My love for you is knowing the sun is going to explode and die. But we can recreate new universes with our touch. Touch is incremental, elemental, our touch holds every raindrop ever fallen, every lightening strike, sunray, snowfall, breeze, wind and hurricane.

Life was made only for this touch.

LOST AND FOUND

It was the meeting of two minds
of 2 people that were lost
who discovered they were not
lost at all.
It was the world around them
that had gone astray
The World used maps like 'work', 'judge'
'hate' and 'blame'
These two did not like to be in those places
there was no escape except to use our
own maps of 'love' 'passion' 'art' and 'poetry'
But we were told:
'There is no place for you here. Tear up
you heart-shaped maps or we will tear
them up for you.'
So we ran away from them
followed our hearts
and
found
each
other

Fragile gun

Fragile gun
Sum of one
That wants to be none

His smile is a bruise
With a laughter that needs to abuse
Nose bent sideways makes strange noises
Silence drowning in a thousand voices
Puffy skin, definition lost
Having a face is too painful
Shit in his pants
But there is a heart beating there
And an unkind mind, a fragile gun
With a million fingers on the trigger
Life has taught him the wrong thoughts to think
But the right stuff to drink
He keeps his eyes closed
He knows how other people look at him
Cider. Communion and destitution
Teeth like dogends
Eyes shine like a sun, yellow with triumphant bile
But no smiles. No smiles.
Flowers are monsters.

Ears like eggcups
The glint in his eyes made of razors
He doesn't look in the mirror any more
His words grate on clouds
His understands laughing graveyards
And why sparrows need helmets and frying pans
And why flowers are still monsters